# Depression: The Demon Within

Lee Zedric Castro

Copyright © 2016 Lee Z Castro

All rights reserved.

ISBN: **1537018884**
ISBN-13: **978-1537018881**

# DEDICATION

My name is Lee Zedric Castro, I am 22 years old and I suffer from Major Depressive Disorder.

That's always the hardest part of our struggle, admitting we have depression. It's the first step towards a big change and the battle to come that will win us the war.

I began writing this book right after my third hospitalization for my depression as it soon became a major road block on my day to day activities. Sitting helplessly in the hospital, dealing with not only the monster hiding behind the door, but also the chemical battle in my body due to the medication, I decided to fight back. I decided that day, while suffering and prepared to surrender and wave the white flag, to stand up and fight back. To remind not only myself but the world and the monster itself that this life is mine, my life will not be run by someone trying to kill, even if that someone is a subconscious part of my mind, it would be run by me.

I wrote this book to not only help myself fight back, but to help inform others, both those who suffer from depression and those who do not. Also to help those who suffer find strength to fight and hopefully help someone win to stay alive.

## Lee Z Castro

I would like to thank my mother and father for their support and understanding on this matter. I am grateful to have a supporting family; most people who suffer from depression do not. This is something that is unacceptable and needs to stop. I would also like to thank my friends for their help over the years fighting this battle.

# Depression: The Demon Within

**Lee Z Castro**

**A warning to the reader:**

**This book is not for the faint of heart, it will reach very dark places in your mind and soul. This book is meant to educate and help those whom suffer with a horrible disease.**

# CONTENTS

|   | Acknowledgments | i |
|---|---|---|
| 1 | A Day in the Life | 1 |
| 2 | Why Fight | 7 |
| 3 | How to Fight | 13 |
| 4 | Victory | Pg # |
| 5 | Honor | Pg # |

# Depression: The Demon Within

Depression is like having a demon walk beside you each and every day. You can feel it breathe on your neck; you see it standing in the corner of every room. No one else can see or hear this monster torturing you each and every day. The reality is, this is your demon to face, yours alone. You see depression is like a war except either you win, or die trying.

People may try to understand how you feel, and you may find solace in speaking with them; however most people cannot comprehend what you are experiencing. Depression is different for everyone, it affects each one of us differently, though the end results may be the same, our demons are different. So even those whom have suffered as we have may still not understand your specific situation, this is something you must remember.

You may not wish to admit you see this dark figure standing there in front of you, staring at you with its red blood shot eyes and razor sharp teeth ready to rip you apart. You may wish to ignore the fact that you have depression that this is simply just a phase which will pass. Don't allow this to happen, don't ignore the demon and allow him to come closer to you each day, closer and closer to pulling you down with him that he may devour you. As I mentioned earlier losing this battle means losing your life.

In this book, we will cover the day to day life in the shoes of the clinically depressed; we will speak of the battle, why to fight, how to fight, the

**Lee Z Castro**

consequences, the end game, and victory. We will also honor those whom have lost their lives in this fight.

# ACKNOWLEDGMENTS

A special mention and thank you to Jeremy, thank you for the support and assistance over the past year regarding my condition, you have been a great help and a great mentor.

# Depression: The Demon Within

**Lee Z Castro**

"Trapped in fear is something I would wish upon my enemies, trapped in ones one mind surrounded by death is something I would wish upon no one."

## 1 A DAY IN THE LIFE

Imagine yourself walking down the street, cold, empty, alone, with one or nothing within reach to comfort you. Do this and you have a small taste into the life of someone suffering from depression.

It is difficult to try and express what the exact feelings are that we feel. They are something that no one else can experience; it's not something modern medicine fully understands. It's the calm cold collective feeling of worthlessness, of solitude, emptiness that clenches your stomach and makes you sick. Such in a way that makes the idea of not living seem like such a paradise.

Your friends tell you they are there for you, and your family states they understand. The doctors tell you the medication is responding well, and that you are making progress. Yet that is not how you feel, your friends seem distant and hard to reach. Your problems seem less important than theirs and you

## Lee Z Castro

wish to not bother them with your issues. Your family looks understanding and caring, but inside you feel they are confused. How can they understand what it is I am going through? The pain, they way it hurts, the endless taunting from the demon standing right in front of me staring at me, reminding me I am truly alone. The doctors grow tired of dealing with the same issues day by day with their patients, at least which is how we feel. Like they are clustering together all our problems from each patient into one and they simply try to repair it. We feel as though no true concern is brought to attention on our specific problems. As I mentioned earlier each one of us is different and suffers in our own particular way. The medicine feels like it causes more harm than good, and though they say you are getting better you feel worse with each day. Sure some days we begin to feel better, but that's because the demon has gone away to slumber and we know inside of our self's he will return.

I am not stating all these things to try and scare you, or try and bring this into a dark place. I state this to inform those of you who do not understand, and to relate to those who do, those who suffer each and every day. To show them that there are people out there who understand and that they are not alone.

There are some whom believe our disease is just a choice that we are simply sad or down. I assure you we do not enjoy felling the hands of the demon on our backs pulling us down, holding us back, and whispering in our ears "Just jump..."

# Depression: The Demon Within

We fight each day, from the beginning of our morning, getting out of bed itself is a major challenge. The sheets seem to wrap around us, keeping us from moving. The thought of just laying there and not moving seems so calming, to simply just cut away the world and lay in our own misery. To not let anyone suffer the way we do, to keep to our self's and let the darkness suffocate us and take us away slowly.

If somehow we can fight back and get up from bed comes the next challenge, the challenge of the day actually coming to a start. The thoughts of why do I need to work? What is the point? When I die it will all come to an end anyways. The feelings of worthlessness begin to kick in, thoughts of darkness begin to cloud our mind. We sit there wondering if it is all worth it, worth getting up and showering, worth getting dressed, or even brushing our teeth. Most people with depression lose their interest in self care, including hygiene. When we can finally breathe in the want to get moving begins the next challenge at work.

Sitting at the office may already seem endless and like a prison to most of us, but those of us with clinical depression suffer with something much more dreadful. Sure we may find our work worthless, and they money not enough, and the time a waste of a day, But most of you may feel this way as well. What is different is we feel the cold in the air that sends chills up our spines. We sit there wanting to bash our head into the computer and hope that it will bring this endless suffering to an

## Lee Z Castro

end. The room seems empty and the conversations are silent and pointless, joy has fled from the world.

When the day has ended we come home, and relive the same questions as we did the morning before we left. Some of us cry and wish the hurting would stop, yet nothing has caused us physical pain. Some of us contemplate way to harm our selves, and even the extreme of ending our lives.


That is a day in the shoes of a Clinically Depressed person.

# Depression: The Demon Within

**Lee Z Castro**

**"Would the world love me ever more so if I could only smile?"**

## 2 WHY FIGHT

I am not going to sit here and tell you I have never hit rock bottom. I am not going to sit here and tell here and tell you I have never tried to end it all, surrender and lose the war. Then I would be a liar, and if there is anything I will not do to you is lie within my own knowledge.

To many of us, sitting out on the edge of a building always sounds like a relaxing motion, a way to let our minds escape. So close to falling, so close to giving in and giving up on it all, yet still breathing, still fighting.

I can't speak from experience on reasons to fight back the demon as many of you can, I can however speak on what I have been told, and what I have heard. Life isn't always about the happy moments, the joy, the smiles. Sometimes life is about the downturns, the tears, the darkness. How we handle these situations makes a huge difference in how we

## Lee Z Castro

handle and enjoy the good times. We cannot let the demon push us around, let us be blinded by his darkness and fall subject to his deceit. It may seem like the best option, to give in and let the emptiness inside our hearts and soul out. To let it simply fly away, as we lay there breathless watching joyous to finally let it all come to an end.

You see depression is your enemy, the one you have faced your whole life. Your true advisory, the one that has always been there and will never just walk away. Constantly bullying you and pushing you to the wall. Enough is enough, you must push back, you must say no!

There is no greater strength than that of a person who fights for something they believe in, if you truly believe in bettering yourself, than do it. Fight back the demon with all that you have inside you, all your power, and will. You must remember all the joy you have had in your life that make it worth going another day. The smallest things make the biggest difference, from your first love, first kiss, your family vacation to where ever it may have been. The first time you drove a car, any moment you can fathom that brought you joy. Yes maybe your depression has clouded these memories and yes perhaps you have more darkness inside you than joy, but somewhere deep inside there is at least one small memory that is worth fighting for.

Fight for that moment to feel that way once more, to simply smile, to laugh, to love. A breath of fresh air,

# Depression: The Demon Within

and a crisp light rain touching your skin may not be your ideal situation, but to many this in itself would make life worth living if not for only another hour. This is what you need to find, that one thing to bring joy back in your life if even for a moment. To make life worth living even if it is just for a day longer. Do this and you will have the will to fight back, and so the battle will begin.

# Lee Z Castro

# Depression: The Demon Within

**Lee Z Castro**

"Joy is not the only thing in life, there is also pain. Yet one minute of joy is worth a day of pain."

## 3 HOW TO FIGHT

There are many ways I can start this chapter, yet small it shall be, it deserves its own chapter non the least.

Fighting back the demon will not be the simplest task you have tackled. No far from it, this will be one of the most difficult challenges you will face in your life time.

What brings you the most joy in life? Is it the way a puppy runs up to you to play? Is it the way that the sun shines off the water as you sit at the beach? Perhaps it's the sound your children make as they play. Whatever it may be, this is going to be your strongest weapon.

Make sure you see a health care professional, how can direct you into the right method of treatment. They should get you to a psychologist, who will talk with you. Do not be afraid, I know it can be difficult to speak to someone about the demon, but this is the best person who can help you accomplish victory. They will do a combination of the following or simply just one over the other. The first option would be medication; most clinical depression is based off of a chemical imbalance in the brain. The medicine will assist you in getting your mind back, getting control again, pushing away that demon into the shadows and bringing out the light.

The next option is going to be therapy, which will be just as if not more affective then the medication, and is ever so much more important to stick with and follow through on.

If ever I convey anything with you, may it be this. The medication and therapy are to help you; they are for you to better yourself. To fight back the darkness that is talking over your body. The demon slowly dissipates as time goes on and you continue the treatments. Remember the small joy that the memory from earlier brings you, and continue with your treatment, be strong, be determined, be free.

Don't be afraid to ask for help, to seek assistance, if a medication isn't working tell someone. I know it is hard to talk, and I know you do not want everyone to know what you are suffering through, but you must make it though. If your therapist isn't helping, don't just stop going, get another one. Call a friend, fight

# Depression: The Demon Within

each battle one step at a time. Don't try to conquer the world in one step; it would be too much even for you. Remember that the only thing that matters is your health, I understand at this moment other people may seem more important to you than yourself, but you cannot allow this.

If you are inpatient at a facility for your treatment, do not freak-out. This is normal, and more than usual. In my opinion it is the best way to receive the top care, at all times of day. Don't go crazy, thinking you will never get out, they will let you out when you are in a better place. Better to be there than wanting to kill yourself, in a place where you can.

**Lee Z Castro**

# Depression: The Demon Within

# Lee Z Castro

"Don't let your sorrow get in the way of your happiness"

# Depression: The Demon Within

## 4 VICTORY

What is victory? Is it winning the race, or simply finishing it?

In our case victory against the demon depression, is many things. It is your first good day after weeks of darkness and despair. It is the first smile after months. Its waking up in the morning and not have to fight to get up. Its working towards a goal, its achieving goals you made for yourself. Your depression is not something that may just disappear from your life for good. It is however though something that can be controlled, and maintained with proper medication and therapy, as well as a positive attitude and direction.

If you can accomplish living each day, one day at a time with only minimal disruption by your depression, you have won! You have succeeded. The war is over and you are the true champion. Congratulations. Don't stop there otherwise the demon will return, keep up with your medication and therapy. It will keep you from setting the world on fire.

To those whom do not suffer from depression, stay positive, help create a positive environment for your friend/family or lover. Don't be afraid to try and support him/her. Create a friendly environment, stay

# Lee Z Castro

positive and supportive.

# Depression: The Demon Within

## Lee Z Castro

"I have finally began to feel better, and the world seems so much clearer."

# Depression: The Demon Within

## 5 HONOR

This chapter holds a very dear place in my heart, in this chapter we will discuss and honor those whom have lost the war against the demon.

As horrible as this is going to sound, over 3,000 people a day around the world commit suicide. That's over one million per year, or one every forty seconds. Without proper support and education on the matter, depression and suicide numbers will continue to rise. This is unacceptable, Those numbers are more than the population of some small countries. Imagine a entire country just committing suicide, It's horrible.

As I mentioned earlier I am no Stanger to suicidal attempts nor am I ashamed to admit I have been in horrible mental depressed moods. Yet I have only ever dealt with one persons suicide whom was close to me, my best friend James. After his suicide I was torn apart, I then slowly realized life moved on. That's one of the tools that helps me fight my depression, knowing that even if I die and let it all end the world continues, it doesn't end, my problems don't disappear. They become someone else's, and I burden them with my death. Suicide is not the best option, I know sometimes it feels like the only one, but keep in mind those whom it affects after.

I dedicate this short story to the people who have lost their lives to the battle against depression.

## ABOUT THE AUTHOR

**Lee Zedric Castro, is a freelance Author and sales consultant. He enjoys writing, swimming, and hikes. He enjoys spending time with his family and friends. To this day Lee has a unconfirmed number of suicide attempts, and fights depression daily.**

www.ingramcontent.com/pod-product-compliance
Lightning Source LLC
Chambersburg PA
CBHW021448170526
45164CB00001B/429